Intermittent Fasting

I0146626

The Complete Guide to Boosting Energy, Resetting Your
Metabolism, and Shedding Pounds

(Guide To Sustaining Your Weight Loss)

Spencer Hargreaves

TABLE OF CONTENT

Chapter 1: Determining Your Optimal Intermittent Fasting Strategy

There are numerous available intermittent fasting plans. After selecting one, I strongly advise you to conduct your own research by reading the plan's author's original text. I have a great deal of respect for these authors, and every book on the list has influenced the way I think about intermittent fasting and its effectiveness. I have personally tried every intermittent fasting regimen imaginable. However, I never considered it a lifestyle, so I would only adhere to a plan for a short time before giving up. The entire tangled story is detailed in Appendix A, if you read my account. As soon as I learned about intermittent fasting, I knew it was the solution for me, but I never committed or followed through until 202 8 , when I was at my lowest point. Once I decided I didn't want to continue riding the weight-gain roller coaster, I was prepared to commit. After realising that intermittent fasting was not merely a diet but a way of life, I experimented until I discovered what worked best for me.

There are two basic types of intermittent fasting strategies: those that are followed daily (called "eating window" approaches) and those that are followed a certain number of times per week (called "up/down day" approaches).

Which intermittent fasting method is the most effective? It is the one that gives you a sense of control and can be adopted as a long-term way of life. It is essential to realise immediately that intermittent fasting is a lifestyle. It's not something you start today and stop when you reach some arbitrary "target weight." A DIET is something you begin and then abandon. As previously stated, intermittent fasting is not a diet but rather a lifestyle. Before I get into the specifics of an eating window approach versus an up/down day approach, I want to revisit the topic of hormones. You may recall from the insulin chapter that insulin determines whether fat is burned or stored. If you keep your body's insulin levels as low as possible, you can burn fat. When insulin levels are elevated, the body tries to store fat. Insulin is the hormone you must comprehend if you wish to lose weight and maintain the loss permanently. However, insulin is not the only hormone that influences your results.

Chapter 2: How Body Fat Is Stolen & Burned

Intermittent fasting has been demonstrated to be an effective method for weight loss and fat burning. But how exactly does it operate? Prior to delving into the inner workings of IF, it is essential to comprehend a few crucial aspects.

Your hormones play a role in the utilisation and storage of energy by your body. Either your body is expending or storing energy. There is no in-between. What does it suggest? If you are not burning glucose (sugar), your body stores it as glycogen or fat. Does this imply that you should engage in regular exercise? No, in a nutshell. 2 0% to 2 10 % of weight loss is attributable to exercise (more on later). The body expends energy in a number of different ways. Even while sitting still and doing nothing, your body uses energy to perform essential functions.

Both RMR and BMR refer to this. However, even if your cells are consuming energy and glucose, any surplus will be stored. This is considered to be a storage state. Wait! If we store sugar or burn it, we should eat less and exercise more to lose weight, according to logic. It seems easy. If you are reading this, it is likely that you have attempted this strategy without success. You initially saw results, but then they stopped or you regained the weight when you returned to your normal routine. Therefore, how can I lose weight? We need to know two things to gain a clearer understanding:

2 . how glucose (sugar) is stored, utilised, and burned.

How do hormones play a role in this?

How do we store energy?

There are two ways for the body to store energy: glycogen and fat. Food (yum) is broken down into various macronutrients during digestion. After being absorbed into the bloodstream, these macronutrients are transported throughout the body to our cells, which perform a variety of functions. For instance, carbohydrates are converted into glucose (sugar), which is absorbed by the blood and transported to the cells for energy use. Glycogenesis, on the other hand, is the process whereby excess glucose in the bloodstream (high blood sugar) is converted into glycogen and stored. The body can only store so much glycogen. Through a process known as lipogenesis, excess glucose is converted into fat when the body's glycogen stores are full.

How is power utilised?

When our cells require more energy than our bloodstream can provide, glycogen is converted back into glucose through a process known as glycogenolysis (low blood sugar). Our glycogen reserves are gradually depleted to restore normal blood sugar levels. When fat stores are depleted, lipolysis is the process by which fat is broken down into energy. Wahoo! We are now burning fat!

Hormones

Hormones, which are commonly associated with mood, also play a significant role in your ability to shed pounds. Multiple stimuli induce their secretion from various glands. For instance, when blood sugar levels rise, the pancreas secretes insulin. We will discuss the most influential hormones on weight loss.

Insulin Trigger: When blood sugar levels rise, insulin is produced.

Purpose: Method for reducing blood sugar: Insulin facilitates the transport of glucose into cells for use as fuel. Any excess is transported to the liver, where insulin stimulates glycogen synthesis by initiating glycogen production.

When you eat, your blood sugar will rise. As a result of this rise, insulin will be secreted. This is common and essential! However, consistent overeating and pointless consumption of starches results in sustained glucose spikes and increased insulin production. Insulin's primary function is to promote storage, so its constant presence in the bloodstream indicates that storage is occurring. Insulin resistance is a condition that can develop if this path is followed for an extended period. Consequently, insulin is less effective because our body has developed an immunity to it. To combat the current high blood sugar levels, more insulin must be released. As a result of the elevated insulin levels in your blood, your liver will produce glycogen and fat more rapidly than ever before!

Glucagon Released when blood sugar levels fall Method for raising blood sugar: Glucagon causes the liver to convert glycogen back into glucose for the bloodstream. Glucagon stimulates adipose tissue, or fat tissue, to break down fat stores in the bloodstream.

Glucagon acts in opposition to insulin, as is evident. This naughty boy's presence in your bloodstream will help your body transition into an energy-burning state.

Leptin Trigger Fat cells secrete leptin. More leptin is delivered in proportion to the number of fatty cells present.

By regulating hunger, satiety, and appetite, leptin contributes to the maintenance of a healthy weight.

Your leptin levels are correlated with your body fat percentage. With increasing body fat, the amount of leptin in the blood increases. Less body fat will result in less leptin in the bloodstream.

During weight loss, Leptin levels will decrease due to the loss of body fat. Consequently, you begin to eat more. If you know this, you'll understand why losing weight sometimes makes you want to eat a horse. Similar to insulin, resistance to leptin can develop in the body. Even if you have a large amount of body fat, leptin will not prevent you from eating because the extra leptin in your bloodstream can cause your body to develop immunity. This may be caused by overeating and the hormonal imbalance mentioned earlier.

Chapter 3: Breakfast Is Not Necessary In The Morning

Breaking your fast is the sole purpose of breakfast. a break for fasting Regardless of when you consume breakfast in the future, it will be considered your first meal of the day. I consume breakfast, for instance, between 2 :00 and 2:00 p.m. Most people find it easier to adhere to 2 6:8 when they begin their eating window later in the day. The opposite is true. Choose a window that appeals to you. Don't fret if you dislike eating in the morning; it is not the reason you cannot lose weight.

According to a study, intermittent fasting does more than just burn fat. When our metabolism changes, both the brain and the body are affected. The New England Journal of Medicine published research demonstrating a variety of health benefits associated with intermittent fasting. It results in a leaner body, a sharper mind, and a longer lifespan.

Several processes that occur during intermittent fasting can protect internal organs from chronic diseases such as inflammatory bowel disease, cardiovascular disease, type 2 diabetes, cancer, and age-related neurodegenerative disorders.

Here are the benefits of intermittent fasting revealed thus far by scientific research:

Diabetes type 2 and obesity. Intermittent fasting is an effective method for adults to lose weight. Fasting can help reduce levels of fasting insulin, fasting glucose, and leptin, as very well as levels of adiponectin and insulin resistance, which is extremely beneficial for individuals with type 2 diabetes. Some studies have found that the majority of patients who engage in intermittent fasting under a physician's supervision require less insulin therapy.

It is important to note that the long-term effects of intermittent fasting have not yet been conclusively established, but current research suggests some intriguing short-term benefits, which I have outlined below.

2 6

It is well-established that the quantity of food consumed has a far greater impact on weight loss than the frequency or timing of meals. In contrast, intermittent fasting may help you maintain a calorie deficit, resulting in weight loss.

However, the fact that you are intermittently fasting does not mean you are in a calorie deficit. Even when they limit the duration of their meals, some individuals still struggle to maintain a healthy calorie intake.

It has been shown that calorie restriction reduces body weight and visceral fat, but maintaining a healthy caloric deficit for extended periods can be difficult. Intermittent fasting is regarded as an effective method for weight loss, as recent human studies reveal significant reductions in body weight and visceral fat.

Weight loss through intermittent fasting may be attributable to factors other than calorie restriction. Fasting-induced physiological changes, such as decreased insulin and leptin levels, may result in greater weight loss than calorie restriction alone.

Ultimately, long-term weight loss requires more than just calorie restriction through methods such as intermittent fasting. Our ability to lose and maintain a healthy weight is influenced by our lifestyle, stress levels, and sleep schedule, among other variables.

Intermittent fasting can be utilised to aid in weight loss, which may compromise other fasting benefits.

2 8

By decreasing levels of leptin, a hormone produced by fat cells to control appetite, and boosting levels of adiponectin, a hormone involved in glucose and lipid metabolism, intermittent fasting and weight loss may help reduce fasting blood glucose and increase insulin sensitivity.

People who intermittently fasted had lower blood glucose levels in a number of trials in which fasting was used as a weight-loss intervention and method for maintaining a healthy weight, which is an important factor in the management and prevention of diabetes.

These potential benefits may be driven primarily by reductions in body weight and body fat percentage as a result of calorie restriction induced by intermittent fasting, despite evidence indicating that intermittent fasting has a positive effect on blood sugar levels overall.

Intermittent fasting may help people with and without diabetes lose weight and improve their glycemic control and insulin sensitivity.

If you consume a nutritious diet during non-fasting periods, your cholesterol levels may improve after intermittent fasting.

Intermittent fasting has been shown to improve lipid profiles by lowering total cholesterol, LDL (low-density lipoprotein), and triglyceride levels in both healthy and overweight individuals.

2 10

Because the majority of studies on the effects of intermittent fasting on cholesterol have focused on those fasting for Ramadan, intermittent fasting may be an effective dietary method for lowering cholesterol; however, more research is required to determine the differences between short-term and long-term metabolic changes associated with fasting.

Consider adopting healthy lifestyle habits, such as exercise and a diet low in saturated and trans fats and high in fibre, if you have high cholesterol.

Intermittent fasting may help protect human hearts by lowering the risk of heart disease and facilitating recovery after a heart attack, although most of the evidence comes from animal studies.

Human trials have demonstrated that intermittent fasting reduces risk factors associated with an increased risk of heart disease, such as:

Bringing down blood pressure

Reducing blood lipid and cholesterol levels regulating glucose levels in the blood

Reducing inflammatory markers including C-reactive proteins and cytokines.

In addition to lowering your resting heart rate, the calorie deficit and metabolic changes caused by intermittent fasting may also help reduce your resting heart rate (HR). Vary your heart rate to enhance vasodilation and blood circulation.

While this may appear promising, humans do not always respond in the same way as animals to these therapies, and additional research on humans is required to understand the 2 6

role of intermittent fasting in cardiovascular disease. Additionally, the quality of your diet is essential for heart health.

The best way to maintain heart health is to consume a diet rich in nutrient-dense whole foods, such as whole grains, fruits, vegetables, and quality meats.

By activating our immune systems, our bodies experience inflammation as part of the process of fighting off harmful pathogens or recovering from injuries.

However, inflammation can become harmful if it persists for an extended period of time. Chronic inflammation occurs when the immune system remains activated in response to what it perceives as a threat. Chronic inflammation contributes to the development of atherosclerosis, heart disease, osteoporosis, and even diabetes.

It has been demonstrated that intermittent fasting reduces levels of pro-inflammatory markers such as homocysteine, interleukin 6, and C-reactive protein, which all contribute to the development of these chronic diseases.

Consuming anti-inflammatory foods or adhering to a strict anti-inflammatory diet or auto-immune protocol (AIP) may also reduce inflammation in the body.

Although fasting may have some health benefits, examining the quality of our meals and lifestyle can assist us in developing healthy habits.

Chapter 4: What Precisely Is Intermittent Fasting?

Fasting has been practised for centuries for a variety of reasons, including improving health, extending life, and religious practise. Consequently, fasting is not merely a passing fad; it is mentioned in the sacred texts of some of the world's most prominent religions, as very well as by eminent philosophers and great thinkers who all attest to the efficacy of intermittent fasting.

The difficulty of determining when to eat presents itself to anyone who has attempted to lose weight. Fasting provides answers to this and numerous other questions.

Have you considered incorporating fasting into your daily routine? The length of the fast varies based on the individual and the reason for observing it. Consider a situation in which you eat dinner late one evening, go to bed, and wake up infrequently to eat during the night. The first meal of the day is breakfast, which is consumed upon awakening. You have just ended a fast that you began the previous evening. It occurs nearly daily.

Additionally, fasting enhances our ability to respond, think, and complete tasks. How do you feel following a reasonably substantial meal? You will likely feel exhausted, tired, sluggish, and unable to think clearly, and you will desire to lie down and sleep.

However, intermittent fasting to reset your body's system and eliminate excess weight and impurities may not be beneficial for everyone. Consult your physician before beginning a fasting programme if you have serious health issues or are not in adequate physical condition. This reconstructed eating pattern must be distinguishable from periodic diet fads. It should be emphasised that this is a method for scheduling meals months in advance.

Intermittent fasting is a popular dietary method that is being studied in laboratories. There may be several benefits to calorie or meal restriction, including the potential for weight loss and a decreased risk of developing certain diseases. However, more research is required to support the effects of intermittent fasting on the health of older individuals.

Alternating between fasting and regular mealtimes, intermittent fasting is an eating strategy. Intermittent fasting focuses solely on when to eat, whereas most diets emphasise what to eat.

During intermittent fasting, you only consume food during the allotted hours. Your body can burn fat if you fast for a set period of time each day or consume only one meal a few times per week. Moreover, scientific evidence suggests that there are health benefits.

When you intermittently fast, you skip all or some meals for a predetermined period before resuming your normal eating habits.

Why hurry?

When we fast, our insulin and blood sugar levels decrease significantly, while our human growth hormone levels increase dramatically. Even though the original purpose of fasting was to aid in weight loss during times of food scarcity, this practise is still prevalent today. Fasting makes fat-burning simple, efficient, and straightforward.

Some people choose to fast because it may increase their metabolism. This type of fasting is beneficial for the treatment of numerous diseases and health conditions.

Fasting is a great method for saving one's life. According to another study, fasting may protect against Alzheimer's, cancer, type 2 diabetes, and cardiovascular disease. Individuals who choose intermittent fasting because it fits their lifestyle make up a separate group. For instance, your life will become easier as you prepare fewer meals.

Chapter 5: Cycles Of Fasting, Labor, And Nursing

Fasting is not advised during pregnancy. Intermittent fasting has been associated with a reduced risk of type 2 diabetes, a heightened metabolism, and weight loss, but it can also cause dangerously low blood sugar levels in pregnant women. In addition to the natural drop in blood pressure that occurs during pregnancy, low blood sugar can cause dizziness and fainting.

Fasting during pregnancy is inadvisable. Intermittent fasting is unsafe for pregnant women because they frequently require an extra evening snack before bedtime or need to eat immediately after waking up, especially in the latter stages of the second trimester.

All women, but especially those who begin their pregnancies underweight or at a healthy weight, should pay close attention to their dietary intake throughout pregnancy (many pregnant women are advised to add about 6 00 more calories per day).

Due to the high nutrient content of breast milk, which is essential to the development of the infant, breastfeeding mothers should avoid long fasts. Fasting during pregnancy may affect the quantity and quality of the mother's milk. Despite the lack of strong medical warnings or scientific evidence against it, women who are breastfeeding are advised not to fast.

Carbohydrates and Body Mass

Low-carbohydrate, high-protein diets may have some short-term weight loss advantages. However, when it comes to preventing weight gain and chronic complaints, carbohydrate quality is significantly more important than carbohydrate quantity.

Mulled, refined grains and the foods made from them, such as white rice, white chuck, white pasta, and repurposed breakfast cereals, are high in casily digestible carbohydrates. Also potatoes and sticky beverages. This is referred to scientifically as having a high glycemic index and glycemic load. Similar foods cause rapid increases in blood sugar and insulin, which, in the short term, can induce hunger and lead to overeating and, in the long term, increase the risk of obesity, diabetes, and heart disease.

For example, in the diet and life change study, participants who increased their consumption of sugary beverages

The consumption of French feasts, potatoes and potato chips, sticky drinks, and meliorated grains resulted in incremental weight gain over time: 6 ,8 ,2 ,6 ,2 ,0, and 0.6 pounds every four years, respectively. People whose consumption of these foods was reduced gained less weight.

Cheese and Weight

The U.S. dairy industry has aggressively promoted the weight- loss benefits of milk and other dairy products, largely based on the results of short-term studies it has funded. However, a recent analysis of nearly 10 0 randomised trials finds little evidence that dairy or calcium consumption aids in weight loss. In addition, most long-term follow-up studies have not found that dairy or calcium protect against weight gain, and one study in adolescents has found a link between high milk intake and an increased body mass index.

A recent study from the Harvard School of Public Health found that people who increased their yoghurt consumption gained less weight; however, increases in milk and garbage consumption did not appear to promote weight loss or gain. The beneficial bacteria in yoghurt may have an effect on weight control, but additional research is required.

There is sufficient evidence that sticky beverages increase the risk of weight gain, obesity, and diabetes. A systematic review and meta-analysis of 88 studies reveal "clear associations between consumption of soft drinks and increased sweet intake and body weight." A more recent meta-analysis estimates that the body mass index of children and adolescents increases by 0.08 units for every fresh 2 2-ounce serving of sweet alcoholic beverage consumed per day.

Another meta-analysis reveals that adults who regularly consume sugary beverages are 26 percent more likely to develop type 2 diabetes than those who consume sugary beverages infrequently. Emerging evidence also suggests that a high intake of sticky beverages increases the risk of heart disease. Sticky vegetables, like refined grains and potatoes, are high in rapidly-digestible carbohydrates. According to research, liquid carbohydrates are not as filling as solid carbohydrates, and people do not consume fewer calories to compensate for the extra calories.

Given that children and adults are consuming ever-increasing amounts of sugary beverages in the United States, these findings are alarming. In the 2 970s, sugary beverages contributed about 8 percent of daily caloric intake, but by 2002 , they contributed about 9 percent of calories. Recent data indicate that on any given day, fifty percent of Americans consume some type of

210 percent consume at least 200 calories from sugared beverages, and 10 percent consume at least 10 67 calories, which is equivalent to four barrels of sugary soda.

The good news is that research on children and adults has also demonstrated that limiting sugary drinks can lead to weight loss.

Chapter 2 : Diverse Methods Of Fasting

There are numerous types of fasts, making it easy to find one that fits your lifestyle.

Below are some of the most prevalent forms of fasting:

Consuming only water for a predetermined period of time constitutes water fasting.

time.

Juice fasting refers to the practise of consuming only fruit or vegetable juice for a predetermined period of time.

Occasional fasting is the temporary restriction of food intake.

hours to a few days at a time, while a normal diet is resumed on other days.

days.

The diet is restricted to no animal products or caffeine for a predetermined period of time.

Calorie restriction

Several days per week, calorie intake is restricted. Within these categories, the number of specialised fasts continues to rise. There are several subcategories of intermittent fasting, for instance.

10 -day fast

Five days per week, consume a regular diet, and two days per week, fast. According to the 10 :2 diet, you should consume a normal diet for five days of the week, followed by two days of fasting. You could, for instance, choose to abstain from food on Monday and Tuesday and eat normally the other days of the week. You can think of it as a single 710 -hour fast per week. For example, eat dinner on Monday at 7 p.m. and don't eat again until breakfast on Thursday morning.

a time-restricted/restricted daily fast

This involves consuming all of your daily meals within a 8 - to 2 2-hour window. You could decide to consume your meals and calories, for example, between 8 a.m. and 6 p.m. It refers to consuming fewer calories during daylight hours. Time-restricted eating is advantageous if you consume your meals before sundown. This not only helps break bad habits such as late-night snacking, but it also improves sleep and blood sugar regulation.

Time-restricted eating can reduce blood sugar levels, improve insulin sensitivity, and reduce blood pressure.

Normalize your eating, but limit your daily eating window to eight hours. For example, skip breakfast and eat lunch at 2 2 a.m. and dinner at 7 p.m.

One-meal-a-day (OMAD) (OMAD)

This involves consuming a single meal containing the entire day's caloric intake within one to two hours. A small study found that type-2 diabetics who fasted for 28 hours three times per week and consumed only dinner on those days no longer needed insulin. In addition, this fasting strategy led to an improvement in HbA2 c, BMI, and waist circumference.

Chapter 6: Reduces blood levels of cholesterol and triglycerides

In addition to improving heart health, fasting can reduce blood cholesterol and triglyceride levels. One study found that alternate-day fasting led to a reduction in these markers, which are important indicators of the risk of heart disease.

Another study found that intermittent fasting in conjunction with a healthy diet improved cholesterol and triglyceride control in comparison to a healthy diet alone.

In addition to rapid weight loss and enhanced fat-burning, intermittent fasting can improve heart health by lowering cholesterol and triglyceride levels.

The levels of cholesterol and triglycerides in our blood are significant markers of heart disease risk, so a reduction in these markers can result in improved heart health.

While most conventional diets stipulate which meals to consume and which foods to avoid, one of the most enticing aspects of the Intermittent Fasting diet is that no foods are forbidden. During the feasting period, you may typically eat whatever you please. Caloric restriction (and its benefits) can be accomplished without sacrificing your favourite foods.

There are numerous diets available, many of which claim to promote weight loss and good health. As a result, it may be challenging to locate one that works. The IF diet is a trendy diet that has gained popularity in recent years. The majority of traditional diets will specify which foods to consume and which to avoid. There is no restriction on the types of foods that may be consumed on an IF diet. This is one reason why some people find it more appealing. Let's compare intermittent fasting to several of the most popular diets.

Calories: Numerous diets require individuals to track or at least consider the number of calories they consume. On a time-restricted intermittent fasting regimen, it is possible to consume the necessary number of calories within the allotted eating time. A person following a time-restricted IF diet will typically have a 6- to 8-hour window in which to consume food. Alternate-day fasting indicates that a person would not consume any food on certain days. This suggests that the calorie intake will fall below the USDA's recommendations. Alternate-day fasting, on the other hand, is a superior method for individuals who consume too many calories to reach their weekly calorie goals.

One of the most appealing aspects of an intermittent fasting (IF) diet is the freedom to consume any food. There are no recommended food categories in intermittent fasting plans, so participants are free to consume whatever they wish. This differs from conventional diets, which tend to restrict certain foods while encouraging the consumption of others. This may be appealing to some, but there is a drawback. Typically, there are no healthy food recommendations included with an IF diet. This indicates that those who regularly consume processed foods are more likely to continue doing so in the future. A person who continues to consume an unhealthy diet while intermittently fasting may not experience the same health and weight loss benefits as those who consume a healthy diet while fasting.

Convenience:

When it comes to dieting, the most common reason people fail is because the diets they adhere to are incompatible with their lifestyle. With intermittent fasting, a person may still consume whatever they desire; the only restriction is the day or time they consume. This generally makes the diet easy to adhere to. Other diets may involve meal planning and grocery lists to facilitate adherence. Those who can control the amount of food they consume may find this to be a very intelligent method for maintaining a healthy lifestyle. Overall, fasting diets have demonstrated promise, particularly for those who struggle to adhere to strict diets. It is essential to remember, however, that intermittent fasting while continuing to make poor food choices does not constitute a healthy lifestyle.

Chapter 7: Adding Intermittent Fasting To Other Diets

As opposed to a diet, intermittent fasting is the practise of eating less frequently and reducing your eating window. You may combine intermittent fasting with any diet you choose, but you must avoid outdated diets such as low-fat or low-calorie diets and instead focus on consuming nutritious foods and minimising carbohydrate intake for optimal results.

2 . Keto Diet and Intermittent Fasting:

The keto diet (ketogenic) was developed approximately a century ago to treat epilepsy in children; it has since gained popularity due to its effectiveness in promoting weight loss. The objective of this diet is to achieve ketosis. Ketosis occurs when the body's primary energy source changes from glycogen to ketone bodies. Your metabolism changes when you stop eating carbohydrates, whether on a ketogenic diet or during an extended fast. According to a study, the ketogenic diet may offer a number of health benefits.

Improveable cardiovascular risk factors include type 2 diabetes, obesity, and HDL cholesterol levels. Although additional randomised, controlled clinical trials are required before precise recommendations can be made, the ketogenic diet has the potential to aid in the treatment of several types of cancer.

Compared to high-carbohydrate diets, a low-carb diet improves type 2 diabetes patients' glycemic control.

Diets with a low glycemic index, such as the ketogenic diet, are effective in treating epilepsy in almost all age groups.

Only a pilot study has examined the effects of the ketogenic diet on polycystic ovary syndrome. Consequently, additional research is required. On the other hand, low-carb diets may be a viable treatment option for this condition.

Integrating the two:

When combining Intermittent Fasting with the ketogenic diet, the standard recommendation is to begin with a low-carb diet and add IF protocols after a few weeks, when the body has adapted to using ketone bodies as its primary source of energy. According to intermittent fasting (IF) and keto experts, it should be easier to reduce your eating window and lengthen your fasting periods when you are already in ketosis. Combining the two diets facilitates weight loss because you consume fewer calories. You no longer only eliminate an entire macro from your diet (due to keto), but depending on your IF programme, you also miss dinners or breakfasts. Despite claims by proponents of the ketogenic diet that it is not a calorie-counting diet, consuming fewer calories aids in weight loss.

People Not permitted with this combination:

The primary drawback of combining intermittent fasting and the ketogenic diet is how restrictive it is. When discussing a healthy weight loss that can be maintained for the remainder of one's life, you are frequently advised that your diet must be sustainable. Rather than a short-term crash diet, you should alter your eating habits permanently.

The ketogenic diet has gained popularity among individuals with type 2 diabetes or pre-diabetes due to evidence that it improves glycemic control and even reduces medication use. Conversely, intermittent fasting may increase the risk of hypoglycemia in people with type 2 diabetes. Those unsuitable for intermittent fasting or the ketogenic diet should avoid combining the two. Anyone who has experienced or is currently experiencing an eating disorder should not attempt intermittent fasting. Women who are pregnant or nursing should avoid intermittent fasting. Consult a physician before beginning intermittent fasting or the ketogenic diet if you have renal disease or any other health condition.

Chapter 8: A Guide to Intermittent Fasting Utilizing the 2 6:8 Fasting Method

The 2 6:8 method of intermittent fasting is the most common and straightforward variant. You will learn everything you need to know about intermittent fasting 2 6/8, including intrustion and imrortant tir, so that you can begin immediately.

For millennia, fasting has been an integral part of numerous world religions and cultures. Today, intermittent fasting is gaining popularity due to its numerous health benefits. There are a number of instances of intermittent fating. The intermittent fasting 2 6/8 method is one of the most common variations.

The 2 6/8 variant of intermittent fasting is a simple, convenient, and sustainable method for losing weight and significantly enhancing overall health.

In this chapter, I will give you a detailed guide to intermittent fasting 2 6/8, explain how it works, and help you determine if it's right for you.

What exactly is 2 6/8 Intermittent Fasting?

The 2 6:8 method of intermittent fasting is both simple and effective. Interval Quick 2 6/8 means restricting the consumption of food and caloric beverages to a fixed eight-hour window per day and abstaining from eating for the remaining 2 6 hours. This fasting regimen can be repeated any number of times, ranging from once or twice per week to daily fasting.

With this method, your daily window for eating is restricted to eight hours. The remaining sixteen hours are spent fasting. Within the 8-hour dining window, you may consume two to three meals. This technique is also known as Leangain Protosol, and fitness expert Martin Berkhan was familiar with it.

The 2 6/8 intermittent fasting method is, in theory, quite simple, as your last meal of the day is dinner and you simply skip breakfast the following day. Interval fast 2 6/8 is a very common form of dieting, especially for those who wish to lose weight quickly and burn fat.

While other diets often have strict rules and exceptions, 2 6/8 interval fasting is extremely simple to follow and can produce rapid weight loss with minimal effort. It is generally considered to be less restrictive and more flexible than other diets, and it can be incorporated into virtually any lifestyle.

In addition to its positive effects on body fat, 2 6/8 interval fasting also improves blood sugar levels and has been shown to increase brain function and longevity.

What Happens in the Bodu During Intermittent Fasting?

The intermittent fasting that follows the 2 6/8 variant is the catalyst for a variety of beneficial changes in your body, right down to the cellular level.

During the fasting period, insulin levels decrease, which increases insulin sensitivity. In addition, your blood sugar level is normalised and you transform into a fat-burning machine.

A keu advantage of short-term dieting is the sustained increase in human growth hormone (HGH), an important hormone involved in sell regeneration that maintains muscle mass during dieting and contributes to the metabolization of body fat.

Short-term fasting also activates the body's self-repair mechanisms, termed autophagy. This ensures that waste and toxins are eliminated from the cells to maintain the health of the body.

Other studies suggest that intermittent fasting is an effective defence against Alzheimer's disease and brain ageing by promoting beneficial changes in specific genes and molecules.

Instructions For Periodic Fasting 2 6/8

Interval fat 2 6/8 is simple, secure, and devoid of issues caused by the need to endure for an extended period of time. To begin intermittent fasting 2 6/8, select an eight-hour window and restrict your food intake to that period.

I would suggest eating between 2 2:00 and 20:00. For many, this is the optimal time to eat at IF 2 6/8, as you will be fasting overnight and will only consume breakfast the following morning. You will have lunch at 2 2:00 slosk as your first meal of the day. So you abstain from food and fast for 2 6 hours.

With a meal window from noon to 8 p.m., you can still have a well-balanced lunch, dinner, and a few small snacks in the afternoon.

Example of daily instructions and schedule for IF 2 6/8:

Your dau starts at 7:00

Immediately following exercise, fat burning is at its peak.

You are permitted to drink coffee for breakfast (no milk, no sugar).

In the morning, you consume a great deal of still water and, if you're feeling a bit hungry, coffee.

At noon, you consume your first meal of the day.

No fast food or readu made rizza! Focus on a nutritious meal (vegetables, salad, meat, fish, etc.).

In the afternoon, you may consume a small snack (such as a handful of nuts, hard-boiled eggs, yoghurt, cereal, etc.).

You will have dinner at approximately 8:00 p.m., which will be your last meal of the day. After that, you will begin a 2 6-hour fast.

The goal of intermittent fasting is to maintain a low insulin level. Every time we consume food, our inulin levels rise.

Milk in soffee, soda, sugaru drinks, ets. All of these increase your insulin levels and should be avoided during your 2 6-hour fast.

When you first begin interval fasting, your body is still accustomed to eating breakfast every day. You will most likely always be hungry when you eat breakfast. This is perfectly normal. Your body has "noticed" which foods are consumed at particular times.

Now that you know breakfast takes longer to appear, your body releases the hunger hormone ghrelin at the time you normally consume breakfast. However, this will subside after a few days, and before you know it, your body will have adjusted and you will no longer feel hungry in the morning.

I've been combining 2 6/8 intermittent fasting with a ketogenic diet for over two years. In fact, I do not feel hungry before 2 6 or 2 8 , despite rising very early.

There are also reorle who prefer to consume food between the hours of 9:00 and 2 7:00. Before the 2 6-hour fasting phase begins, you have time for a hearty breakfast at 9:00 am, a normal lunch around noon, and a light early dinner or snack at 8 :00 pm.

Of course, you must experiment and select the optimal time frame for your career and personal life. The most important fact is that you are fasting for 2 6 hours without eating anything.

Regardless of when you consume your meals, it is recommended that you consume 2-6 small meals and snacks throughout the day. In this manner, you can stabilise your blood sugar and control your appetite.

To maximise the health benefits of intermittent fasting, it is also essential to consume nutrient-dense whole foods and sugar-free beverages during mealtimes. Eating fresh and nutrient-dense foods can assist you in improving your diet and maximising the benefits of intermittent fasting.

Chapter 9: Getting Started With Intermittent Fasting

It is believed that rigorous diet plans have evolved over time. Intermittent fasting focuses solely on when to eat, whereas most diets emphasise what to eat.

During intermittent fasting, you only consume food during the allotted hours. If you fast for a set period of time each day or consume only one meal a few days per week, your body can burn fat. Moreover, scientific research indicates that there are health benefits. It is safe to say that humans have practised intermittent fasting for centuries.

Prior to cultivating crops, early humans were hunters and gatherers who developed the ability to survive without food for extended periods of time. Hunting animals and gathering nuts and berries required considerable time and effort.

TV, the internet, and other forms of entertainment are now accessible in the modern era. In order to watch our favourite television programmes, we stay up later and engage in less productive daytime activities, such as binge eating.

We are blind to the fact that less exercise and more calories can increase the risk of type 2 diabetes, cardiovascular disease, obesity, and other conditions. According to scientific studies, intermittent fasting may be able to buck these trends and improve our quality of life.

Chapter 10: How does intermittent fasting function?

There are numerous ways to practise intermittent fasting, but they all begin with establishing regular eating and fasting windows. You could, for instance, eat only for the first eight hours of the day and then fast for the following eight. Alternately, you can choose to consume only one meal per day, twice per week. Intermittent fasting schedules vary widely. By extending the time until your body has burned off the calories from your last meal and begins to burn fat.

Chapter 11: Working Out During A Fast

Exercise is also essential to the success of intermittent fasting. Exercise offers many excellent advantages. It may help with depression and anxiety while allowing you to achieve your aesthetic goals. Exercise will also affect the balance of the hormones described previously. Exercise increases the production of Human Growth Hormone, but accelerates glycogen depletion.

What is the optimal exercise while fasting?

It is a common misconception that prolonged exercise at a constant speed is the most effective way to burn fat. My experience indicates otherwise. Although it has its benefits, I've had far more success with High Intensity Interval Training for both male and female clients when it comes to fat burning and the intermittent fasting lifestyle.

Training with High Intensity Intervals

If fat loss is your goal, particularly if you are 10 0 or older, I recommend this programme. Fast-paced exercises that can be completed in 6 0 minutes make this programme ideal for people with hectic schedules. This can be accomplished utilising bodyweight exercises, barbells, kettlebells, and dumbbells. Typically, I incorporate workouts that target multiple muscle groups. For instance, a row instead of a bicep curl. Rapid bursts of near-maximal effort define the objective.

To obtain the greatest possible benefits from intermittent fasting, you must engage in physical activity. Adopting any form of exercise, be it strength training or aerobics, can expedite your weight loss considerably. Follow along as I demonstrate an intermittent fasting exercise and provide guidance to ensure you're doing things correctly.

Working Out During a Fast

Exercising while fasting is one of the most effective methods for weight loss. Intermittent fasting aids in the accumulation of a calorie deficit, which is exacerbated by the addition of exercise. Without a doubt, this combination is incredibly effective, but you must ensure you're doing everything correctly to preserve lean body mass.

When combining fasting and exercise, there are two factors in particular that must be considered.

How rigorous your workouts are. Alternatively, how many calories do you burn per gym session?

How long your fast will last. The longer you go without food, the greater number of calories you will burn.

You should consider these factors because you don't want to expend an excessive number of calories. Rapid weight loss will inevitably lead to muscle gain, and lean tissue is your ally.

Assume, for the sake of illustration, that you fast for 2 6 hours per day, which is relatively common. A calorie deficit can be created by fasting for 2 6 hours, but it would be less pronounced compared to a 20-hour fast. Therefore, a person who fasts for 2 6 hours per day may be able to exercise more vigorously than the latter.

Exercise Timing

During the fasting phase is the optimal time to exercise. If your workouts are of high volume and intensity, you should be prepared to break your fast immediately afterward. Although not required, this is primarily to ensure that your body receives some protein.

There are two foolproof methods for determining the best time to exercise. You can exercise either immediately prior to the meal that breaks your fast or shortly after your final meal of the day.

Both options ensure that your body receives sufficient protein to repair exercise-related damage. The first occurs immediately after a meal, while the second occurs just prior to a meal. Regardless of which option you choose, I recommend breaking your fast shortly after your workout. This replenishes your body with many calories and much-needed protein.

The most effective method for establishing a routine is to exercise in the morning. After your last meal of the day, you will rest and exercise the following morning. By now, it should be time to break your fast, and you may enjoy a delicious meal after your workout.

Fasting Exercise Format

Intermittent fasting is often misunderstood, but when combined with physical activity, it is actually beneficial. As previously mentioned, you must ensure you have a plan to not only lose weight but also maintain muscle mass.

Resistance Exercise:

This involves resistance training. For optimal results, consider an upper/lower workout split or a PPL programme. Attempt to lift weights three to six times per week to build and maintain muscle mass. Below is an example of a highly beneficial three-day weight training programme.

Monday: Push (Back, Biceps) (Biceps, Back)

Tuesday is Free

Pull (Quads, Hamstrings, Glutes, Calves) on Wednesday (Quads, Hamstrings, Glutes, Calves)

Thursday: Holiday

Legs (chest, triceps, shoulders) on Friday (Chest, Triceps, shoulders)

Weekend: Off

Choose a programme for specific exercises, but the above outline is an example of balanced training. The volume and intensity of your workouts will be greater if you exercise three times per week than if you exercise more frequently.

Cardio:

Low-intensity steady-state cardio yields the most beneficial results. This exercise is exemplified by incline walking on a treadmill. If you're training quickly, you're already burning a lot of calories, so you shouldn't perform HIIT or anything else that requires a lot of energy.

Recommended treadmill settings for performing cardio while fasting:

Incline: 6.10 - 2 2.10 %

Between 2.710 and 6 .610 mph

These settings produce a brisk walking pace that burns between 200 and 6 00 calories per half-hour. Obviously, the number of calories you burn is dependent on the incline and pace you choose.

Tips For Fighting Hunger

After a long fast, I understand that sometimes you just want to consume everything in your refrigerator. In reality, the sensation of hunger (which is actually your appetite) will increase if you combine exercise. However, that should not intimidate you, as there are numerous ways to control your hunger when you have a few hours left.

Shorten your fasting window — Perhaps you began with 20-hour fasts because you were overly ambitious. If so, begin slowly and work your way back down to 2 6-hour fasts. Once you're comfortable, you can gradually increase the time, but 2 6 hours is an excellent starting point.

Again, this tip is not universally applicable.

Soon after your last meal, retire to bed. The most effective method for avoiding late-night cravings is to go to bed early. Typically, this entails sleeping immediately after your last meal. You will likely feel less hungry as a result, as you will be awake for less time.

Caffeine — Whether you consume it in the form of black coffee or a calorie-free pre-workout supplement, caffeine is excellent. There may not be a stronger appetite suppressant vitamin. If you are able to consume coffee, it is unquestionably an excellent tool to use during fasting.

Make your last meal the largest - This is entirely up to you, but if you have a busy night ahead, eating a large last meal will keep you full. Obviously, you don't want to overeat, but you should try to fill yourself up with your last meal. This is especially true if you exercise after eating.

Consume a great deal of water - Filling your stomach with water is the most effective way to control hunger. Aim for 68 -2 28 ounces of water per day, and drink a glass of water whenever you feel hungry. Water is your best friend during a fast because it contains zero calories and is excellent for physiological function.

Chapter 12:   The Major Advantages And Disadvantages Of Trying Intermittent Fasting

Intermittent fasting, the trendy health fad involving periods of abstinence from food, offers numerous advantages and disadvantages, just like everything else. Intermittent fasting may improve cognitive function, physique, and disease risk.

There are several disadvantages associated with intermittent fasting, including the potential for health problems, the difficulty of long-term compliance, and the possibility of social consequences. It is nearly impossible to research nutrition and fitness trends without encountering information about intermittent fasting.

It is important to remember that there are numerous ways to implement this type of dietary trend, which entails going a certain amount of time without consuming any calories.

Some individuals recommend following the 2 6:8 diet, which entails not eating for 2 6 hours per day and then consuming all of your daily meals and calories within a fixed eight-hour window. Some recommend the 10 :2 diet, which consists of two days of fasting and consuming no more than 10 00 calories, followed by five days of unrestricted eating. Other forms of intermittent fasting recommend completing a weekly 6 6-hour fast.

There are numerous variations of intermittent fasting, so you can choose the one that works best for you. Pro: Intermittent fasting promotes a healthier physique. As with everything, there are both benefits and drawbacks.

Pro: Intermittent fasting promotes body composition improvement.

Since fasting involves not eating, it seems reasonable to assume that consuming fewer calories than usual will result in weight loss. After consuming all of your stored glucose for fuel during a fast, you may access your fat reserves. When our fat reserves begin to be burned, body fat loss commences.

Intermittent fasting helps to improve body composition by necessitating a calorie deficit, promoting weight loss and reducing body fat, and enhancing our metabolism through its effect on hormones.

Commitment to the Long-Term May Be Difficult

In order to achieve a caloric deficit, intermittent fasting requires that you abstain from eating for a predetermined period of time, followed by a predetermined calorie intake within a predetermined window of time. Due to low energy, cravings, habits, and the discipline necessary to adhere to the precise time frames surrounding your periods of intermittent fasting, long-term maintenance of this extended period of zero-calorie consumption may be challenging.

Due to the amount of self-discipline required to sustain intermittent fasting, it is also difficult to do so for an extended period. It may be challenging to adhere to both sides of intermittent fasting; it is equally important to avoid bingeing when it's time to eat and eating when you shouldn't be fasting.

The researcher and author of "Eat, Stop, Eat," Brad Pilon, recommends acting as if nothing has transpired after breaking your fast. No compensation, no incentives, no special diet, drinks, or medications.

This is necessary for the intermittent fasting process, and ultimately for your own good.

Pro: Intermittent Fasting May Help Prevent and Decrease the Incidence of Illness

According to the Cleveland Clinic, fasting may also aid in diabetes management, cholesterol reduction, and blood pressure reduction. All of these are significant disease-causing risk factors that must be managed.

Contrary to those who adhered to a more conventional, regular daily meal schedule, those who followed an intermittent fasting diet experienced a 9 percent decrease in blood pressure, according to a study conducted by University of Surrey experts.

Another study discovered that intermittent fasting promoted sleep, which in turn decreased blood sugar and inflammation — two major contributors to the development of chronic diseases like diabetes and cardiovascular disease. The vast majority of our social interactions occur over food and drink. You must have the self-control to refrain from indulging while fasting, or you must find other ways to maintain your social life without breaking your fast.

Although difficult, it is achievable.

However, fasting may also be exhausting. While you're fasting, you'll have less energy than usual, so you may feel the need to rest in order to conserve what little energy you do have.

It's a difficult balancing act.

Neurogenesis, which is the "growth and development of new brain cells and nerve tissues" in the brain, is accelerated by fasting. Consequently, memory, attention, mood, and brain function are enhanced.

In addition, going without food stresses the brain and prompts it to take precautions against infections. The body enters a state known as ketosis, which uses fat as fuel to "increase energy and eliminate brain fog," which is said to be the cause.

We've all heard that brain-stimulating puzzles and other activities are good for us, and it appears that fasting's challenges are no exception.

Intermittent fasting may cause hormonal abnormalities in individuals who already lead active lifestyles or were thinner prior to beginning it.

This can lead to irregular menstrual cycles and the potential for reproductive issues in individuals who identify as women. Hormonal imbalances may cause thyroid problems, insomnia, and increased stress in all individuals.

Numerous health benefits of intermittent fasting have been demonstrated, and further research is ongoing. In addition, intermittent fasting may be compatible with certain individuals' notions of a long-term, sustainable diet.

Weight management and maintaining metabolic health are the two primary motivations for intermittent fasting. Metabolic health is a measure of the body's ability to metabolise or digest energy. Frequently, blood pressure, blood sugar, and blood fat levels are used as indicators.

A calorie deficit occurs when your body consumes fewer calories than it requires to maintain its current weight. This may occur when fasting or going without food. Consequently, the majority of weight loss programmes rely on calorie restriction, such as fasting.

Certain forms of intermittent fasting may be just as beneficial for weight loss as other calorie-restrictive diets, if not more so, according to research.

Time-restricted eating patterns, such as the 2 6/8 method, are one form of intermittent fasting that has been directly linked to weight loss. Additionally, the 10 :2 diet and alternate-day fasting may be beneficial.

In addition to helping you burn calories naturally while fasting, intermittent fasting may also help you lose weight by suppressing your appetite and making you feel fuller for longer.

Additional health advantages of the eating pattern include:

Bringing down blood pressure

enhancing glucose management

Mending damaged cells

Maintaining cognitive ability

Could Cause a Permanent Change in Lifestyle

Despite the fact that intermittent fasting may appear daunting and difficult, it is occasionally quite simple. Because fewer meals need to be planned, you may find that fasting simplifies your day.

In addition, it typically does not require calorie tracking, macro monitoring, eating meals you may not normally eat, or avoiding meals you may normally enjoy.

For example, one method of intermittent fasting is to eat dinner early and then sleep in. If you eat your last meal at 8 p.m. and do not eat again until 2 2 p.m. the next day, you have officially fasted for 2 6 hours.

Individuals who typically eat breakfast in the morning or who cannot eat until later in the evening due to work or other obligations may find it difficult to adopt this strategy.

However, this is the normal diet of other people. They might be more inclined to try an intermittent fasting diet.

Combines very well with a diet abundant in nutritious foods.

Intermittent fasting is typically simple to incorporate into your current diet, as it places a greater emphasis on when you consume food than on what you consume.

You will not need to purchase any special foods or alter your regular diet.

If your diet is going very well but you're still looking for ways to improve your overall health, you may want to consider fasting.

Individuals who wish to combine intermittent fasting with resistance training and a high-protein diet, for example, may find it to be quite effective. However, this does not imply that what you consume is irrelevant. Consuming a variety of nutritious foods and avoiding highly processed foods during your eating window will maximise the benefits of intermittent fasting.

Intermittent fasting is frequently used for weight management and metabolic health. The eating plan can reduce blood pressure, blood sugar, and blood fat levels. It also works for some individuals as a healthy, long-term eating plan.

Consequences Of Sporadic Eating

Intermittent fasting is a method for controlling caloric intake and working to improve metabolic health.

Despite the fact that the eating pattern is undoubtedly a component of a balanced diet, it will likely take some getting used to initially. Additionally, intermittent fasting should not be practised by everyone.

Here are some disadvantages you may encounter when beginning an intermittent fasting regimen.

Women could benefit from intermittent fasting less than men do. Intermittent fasting may harm female fertility, according to some animal studies.

People who have a history of eating disorders may want to stay away from intermittent fasting. Fasting is a risk factor for eating disorders, according to the National Eating Disorders Association.

Additionally, those with a history of sadness and anxiety may not be good candidates for the 2 6:8 schedule. According to some studies, calorie restriction might worsen depression over the long run, but it can also have the opposite impact in the short term. To fully comprehend the ramifications of these discoveries, further study is required. For persons who are attempting to become pregnant, are nursing, or are pregnant, 2 6:8 intermittent fasting is not advised.

According to the National Institute on Aging, there is not enough support for any fasting diet recommendations, particularly for older persons.

People should consult their doctor before using the 2 6:8 technique or any other kind of intermittent fasting, particularly if they are on medication or have:

• underlying medical conditions, including diabetes or low blood pressure
• a history of mental health issues or disordered eating

Anyone who is worried about anything or feels any negative effects from the diet should contact a doctor.

Diabetes

Research indicates that the 2 6:8 technique may be useful for preventing diabetes, but those who already have the disease may not be able to use it.

Diabetics of type 2 should not adhere to the 2 6:8 intermittent fasting diet. With the assistance of a physician, certain individuals with type 2 diabetes or prediabetes may be able to attempt the diet.

Before altering their diet, those with diabetes who wish to adopt the 2 6:8 intermittent fasting diet should consult a physician. 2 6:8 intermittent fasting is a common form of intermittent fasting. Weight loss, fat burning, and a decreased risk of contracting certain diseases are all potential benefits.

Compared to other fasting methods, this diet may be easier to adhere to. People who practise 2 6:8 intermittent fasting should focus on consuming fiber-rich whole meals and staying hydrated throughout the day.

The proposal will not benefit everyone equally. If a person has concerns or underlying health issues and wishes to follow the 2 6:8 intermittent fasting diet, they should consult a physician or nutritionist first.

Contradicts Your Instincts Perhaps

Intermittent fasting requires self-control, restraint, and preparation.

Using these strategies to limit your caloric intake within a specific time frame may not be an issue for some individuals, despite the fact that it may seem strange to them. This may be especially true if you frequently eat whenever you feel hungry.

In addition, if you prefer not to adhere to a rigid schedule, you may find intermittent fasting annoying. In addition, if your schedule fluctuates from day to day due to family, work, or other obligations, it may be difficult to adhere to a specific caloric intake period.

When one is not accustomed to fasting, even an eight- or twelve-hour fast may seem excessive. Multiple times per week, it is possible to go to bed hungry. Obviously, it may appear uncomfortable and ultimately untenable. In order to avoid breaking your fast prematurely, it is sometimes necessary to ignore your normal hunger and satiety cues.

This is not to say that you cannot become accustomed to intermittent fasting. After you have become accustomed to intermittent fasting, you may even discover that it reduces your appetite.

After a few months, many people become accustomed to the pattern, and some even begin to enjoy it. However, it is normal to initially anticipate and be aware of hunger and irritation.

Chapter 13: Tips On Maintaining Your Intermittent Fasting Plan

Consuming food is an integral part of living. Not only is eating essential for nourishing the body and maintaining health, but it is also a social activity. Whether you enjoy holiday feasts with family or prefer late-night snacking, studying intermittent fasting may seem like a nuisance. Having a solid plan of attack may, however, position your experience for success. Here are eight suggestions for maintaining an intermittent fasting diet.

Intermittent fasting is not recommended for the faint-hearted. Therefore, it is preferable to have a plan before beginning. Thus, you can remain aware of where you may encounter obstacles and the desire to quit. Here are some suggestions for sticking to an Intermittent Fasting programme:

Start with a fundamental intermittent fasting technique

Beginners should not begin with OMAD (one meal a day) intermittent fasting if that is their primary objective. Select an appropriate starting plan and work your way up to a single daily meal. Start with a 2 8 /2 0 intermittent fasting strategy with a 2 0-hour window for eating, for instance. Finally, you may transition to a more rigorous 2 8/6 regimen, followed by a 20/8 fasting schedule. Taking baby steps towards a larger objective can acclimatise your body and mind to time-restricted eating.

Plan your meals, especially your meal to break your fast.

When people are hungry, their judgement is typically impaired. In fact, this is how the term "hangry" originated. Hunger can cause irritability, so if you don't have a plan in place, you might grab the first item that looks appetising. Do not indulge in office doughnuts or milkshakes on the way home from work.

Plan the meal that will break your fast. Eat at a healthy restaurant, prepare a meal in a slow cooker at home, or carry a handful of nuts in your vehicle to stave off hunger until you can eat a full meal. A strategy will assist you in maintaining an effective intermittent fasting regimen.

When you deviate from your plan, do not throw in the towel.

Note that the phrase states when, not if. There may be circumstances in which you must abandon your intermittent fasting regimen. Life happens. Perhaps you need to make dietary changes for health reasons. Possibly a family emergency makes it impossible to adhere to a time-restricted diet at the moment. Perhaps it's Thanksgiving, and all you want to do is feast for the entire day. Everything is acceptable. Truly!

Give yourself permission to fall off the waggon for a day, a week, or a season. This will give you the mental space to deal with whatever life throws at you. Even if you had no reason to cheat except for the fact that you caved in and ate a brownie before bed, that is acceptable. Simply rise and continue your fasting journey the following day. The beauty of it is that you can move on and start over whenever you're ready.

Find a suitable intermittent fasting strategy for yourself.

Pragmatism dictates that if you adhere to the OMAD diet, your only meal should be dinner. For many, if not the majority, this makes sense. You may rise, go about your day, and anticipate a satisfying dinner to conclude the day. However, avoid allowing typical factors to affect your intermittent fasting regimen. It's acceptable to eat only breakfast or lunch. Some individuals may find it difficult to concentrate at work without a morning meal. Others are able to delay their hunger until lunch, but their inability to eat renders their entire afternoon unproductive.

Do what works best for you, even if it means adopting a different intermittent fasting technique.

If OMAD is difficult (and it is), perform it once per week. Six days later, switch to a different method, such as intermittent fasting 2 8/6. Allow yourself the freedom to create a schedule that complements your lifestyle and circadian rhythm.

Consume copious amounts of water while fasting.

Water is essential for the proper functioning of the human body. It is also essential to rid our bodies of toxins and support the metabolic processes occurring during fasting. Cells are repairing and replacing damaged components, with hydration aiding the process. You may also consume zero- or low-calorie liquids, such as tea, so long as they do not contain added sugars.

Make the most of your pre-fasting meal.

Combine a nourishing dinner with a Fastful bar, which will help your body maximise nutrition and keep you feeling full for longer. Preparing for a successful fasting period will make the period more bearable.

Recognize that your fasting results may vary.

Not everyone has the same body. We all have diverse appearances, varied medical histories, and distinctive lifestyles. If you have a specific goal in mind, such as losing weight or lowering your blood pressure, be patient. One individual may experience rapid weight loss, while another may experience slow weight loss. Enter the fast with an open mind. Know that your body will undergo imperceptible changes, such as cell recycling and improvement of your general neurological health, even if your weight loss is minimal.

Avocado Quesadillas

Ingredients:

- 6 tbsp. of fresh coriander, chopped
- 1/2 cup of sour cream
- 50 inches of flour tortillas
- 1/2 cups of Monterey Jack cheese, shredded
- 1 tsp. of vegetable oil
- 2 avocado (ripe), pitted, peeled and chopped into 1/2 inch pieces
- 4 tomatoes (vine-ripe), seeded & chopped into 1/2 inch pieces
- 2 tbsp. of chopped red onion
- 1/2 tsp. of Tabasco sauce
- 4 tsp. of fresh lemon juice
- salt and black pepper

Directions:

1. Combine the tomatoes, onion, avocado, lemon juice, and Tabasco in a small bowl.

2. Season with salt & pepper to taste.

3. Mix sour cream, salt, coriander, and pepper to taste in a separate small bowl.

4. Brush the tops of the tortillas with oil and place them on a baking pan.

5. 2-8 inches from the flame, broil tortillas until lightly golden.

6. Sprinkle cheese evenly over tortillas and broil until melted.

7. To create 4 quesadillas, spread the avocado mixture equally over 4 tortillas & top each with 1-5 of the remaining tortillas and cheese side down.

8. Cut the quesadillas into four wedges on a chopping board.

9. Serve heated with a spoonful of the sour cream mixture on top of each slice.

Apple Cider Vinegar Limeade Recipe

Ingredients

- 2 cup of ice
- 4 medium lime (juiced)
- Sweetener

- 2 tablespoon of apple cider vinegar
- 2 cup of water

Instructions

- Put all the ingredients together in the cocktail shaker
- Shake it very well to mix them
- Serve over ice